CHEMO DIET C
FOR BEGINNERS

Quick and Easy Anti-Cancer Recipes for Cancer Treatment and Recovery

Merissa O. Hardin

Copyright © 2024 by Merissa O. Hardin

All rights reserved. No part of this publication may be reproduced, distributed, or transmitted in any form or by any means, including photocopying, recording, or other electronic or mechanical methods, without the prior written permission of the publisher, except in the case of brief quotations embodied in critical reviews.

TABLE OF CONTENTS

INTRODUCTION 9
What is a Chemotherapy DIET? 13
Importance of nutrition during chemotherapy 16
Importance of Hydration during Treatment 20
Key Nutrients for Cancer Patients 23
Building a Balanced Meal 27
    Choosing the Right Proteins 27
    Incorporating Healthy Carbohydrates 28
    Including Essential Fats 29
Combating Common Side Effects 30
    Managing Nausea through Diet 30
    Foods to Combat Fatigue 31
    Maintaining Appetite during Treatment 32
Food to Eat and Food to Avoid 33
    Foods to Include 33
    Foods to Avoid or Limit 35
Chapter 1 37
    Breakfast recipes 37
    1. Berry Protein Smoothie Bowl 37
    2. Oatmeal with Almond Butter and Banana Slices 38
    3. Avocado and Tomato Breakfast Toast 39
    4. Coconut and Mango Chia Pudding 40
    5. Spinach and Feta Egg Muffins 41

6. Banana Walnut Breakfast Cookies 43

7. Quinoa Breakfast Bowl 44

8. Cottage Cheese and Pineapple Parfait 45

9. Sweet Potato and Spinach Frittata 46

10. Blueberry Almond Chia Seed Pudding 47

11. Peanut Butter Banana Toast 48

12. Yogurt and Granola Parfait 49

13. Apple Cinnamon Overnight Oats 50

14. Mango Coconut Rice Pudding 51

Chapter 2 52

Lunch Recipes 52

1. Chicken and Quinoa Bowl 52

2. Salmon and Quinoa Salad 53

3. Vegetarian Quinoa Stir-Fry 55

4. Mango Avocado Chickpea Salad 56

5. Turkey and Vegetable Skewers 58

6. Lemon Garlic Shrimp Pasta 59

7. Spinach and Feta Stuffed Chicken Breast 61

8. Cauliflower and Broccoli Soup 62

9. Egg and Vegetable Wrap 64

10. Sweet Potato and Black Bean Chili 65

CHAPTER 3 67

Dinner Recipes 67

1. Salmon and Sweet Potato Skewers 67

2. Baked Lemon Garlic Chicken 68

3. Chickpea and Spinach Curry 70

4. Turkey and Vegetable Skillet 72

5. Mushroom and Brown Rice Risotto 73

6. Lemon Herb Baked Cod 75

7. Vegetable and Lentil Soup 76

8. Shrimp and Broccoli Stir-Fry 78

CHAPTER 4 79

Appetizers and snacks 79

1. Hummus and Veggie Platter 79

2. Greek Yogurt and Berry Parfait 80

3. Avocado and Tomato Salsa with Whole Grain Chips 81

4. Cucumber and Smoked Salmon Rolls 83

5. Edamame and Sea Salt 84

6. Caprese Skewers 85

7. Roasted Red Pepper and White Bean Dip 86

8. Baked Sweet Potato Fries 87

9. Turkey and Cranberry Lettuce Wraps 88

CHAPTER 5 90

Soup and Stews Recipes 90

1. Healing Chicken and Rice Soup 90

2. Vegetarian Lentil and Spinach Stew 92

3. Creamy Butternut Squash Soup 93

4. Salmon and Vegetable Chowder 95

5. Tomato Basil and Chickpea Stew 96

6. Chicken and Vegetable Noodle Soup 98

7. Creamy Broccoli and Cauliflower Soup 99

8. Spiced Lentil and Carrot Soup 100

9. Mushroom and Brown Rice Congee 102

CHAPTER 6 104

Main Dish- Poultry Recipes 104

1. Lemon Herb Baked Chicken 104

2. Turkey and Vegetable Stir-Fry 105

3. Baked Pesto Chicken 107

4. Honey Mustard Grilled Chicken 108

5. Herb Roasted Turkey Breast 109

6. Lemon Garlic Turkey Burgers 110

7. Chicken and Brown Rice Casserole 111

8. Orange Glazed Chicken 113

9. Mango Salsa Turkey Tacos 114

CHAPTER 7 116

Main Dish- Seafood Recipes 116

1. Baked Lemon Garlic Salmon 116

2. Shrimp and Avocado Salad 117

3. Grilled Lemon Herb Swordfish 119

4. Baked Cod with Tomato Salsa 120

5. Lemon Garlic Butter Shrimp Pasta 121

6. Teriyaki Glazed Salmon 123

7. Mango Salsa Tuna Salad 124

8. Cajun Grilled Shrimp Skewers 126

9. Halibut with Roasted Vegetables 127

10. Seared Scallops with Lemon Butter Sauce 129

CHAPTER 8 130

Main Dish- Vegetarian 130

1. Eggplant and Chickpea Curry 130

2. Mushroom and Spinach Risotto 131

3. Sweet Potato and Black Bean Enchiladas 133

4. Quinoa and Vegetable Stir-Fry 135

5. Caprese Quinoa Salad 137

6. Chickpea and Vegetable Curry 138

7. Stuffed Bell Peppers with Quinoa and Black Beans ... 140

8. Pesto Zucchini Noodles with Cherry Tomatoes 141

CHAPTER 9 143

   Conclusion 143

INTRODUCTION

Emma found herself in the calm community of Serenity Hills, facing an unexpected voyage. She was diagnosed with cancer and went on a difficult journey that included rounds of treatment. As the therapies continued, Emma recognized how important diet was for maintaining her body.

Emma began researching a specialized diet intended for patients receiving chemotherapy with the help of her physician and a qualified nutritionist. It wasn't just about the food; it was about nourishment, fortitude, and perseverance.

Emma's mornings began with vivid smoothie bowls loaded with antioxidants and nutrients. Fresh berries, spinach, and a scoop of protein powder combined to make a wonderful smoothie that not only fed her body but also elevated her mood. The rush of flavors became a daily source of joy in her otherwise difficult schedule.

For lunch, Emma chose hearty soups with immune-boosting components. A warm bowl of homemade chicken soup and vegetables became a soothing habit. The warmth engulfed her, bringing peace on the most difficult days. The soup was more than just food; it was a reminder that every spoonful contained healing potential.

As Emma progressed through chemotherapy, she found the joys of vibrant salads and nutrient-dense side dishes. Avocado and tomato salads, quinoa with roasted vegetables, and sweet potatoes were cornerstones of her diet. These recipes not only delighted her taste buds, but also improved her general well-being.

Emma's main courses were carefully designed to incorporate lean proteins and nutritious grains. Her dinners became centered around baked salmon with a variety of herbs, quinoa, and roasted vegetable pilaf, as well as grilled chicken with a citrus sauce. Each bite represented a dedication to health and a little win over the hurdles she faced.

Emma relied heavily on snacks and little nibbles throughout the day. Hummus and veggie platters, Greek yogurt parfaits, and energy-boosting trail mix all supplied the energy needed to go through chemotherapy. Emma learnt that resilience may be found in even the smallest bites.

Desserts became a welcome pleasure, demonstrating that sweetness could be part of a chemo-friendly diet. Berry and Greek yogurt popsicles, banana-oat biscuits, and dark chocolate avocado mousse were guilt-free treats that provided moments of joy throughout the treatment program.

Hydration became a concern, and Emma experimented with infused water recipes and pleasant green smoothies. Staying hydrated helped her body deal with the negative effects of chemotherapy, making the journey more bearable.

Meal planning and preparation were Emma's secret weapon. With weekly meal plans, she assured a consistent supply of nutritious dishes. Her kitchen was transformed into a sanctuary, filled with the aroma of fresh food and the promise of brighter days to come.

Emma found strength in the intentional link between food and healing as she adopted this specialized chemo-friendly diet, in addition to managing the physical hurdles of chemotherapy. The meticulously prepared meals became more than just food; they were Emma's comrades in the fight for her health.

In the heart of Serenity Hills, a story unfolded—one of resilience, sustenance, and the transformational power of a well-planned diet. Emma's story demonstrated that, even in the midst of adversity, one may find courage and solace in the simple act of deciding what to put on the plate.

WHAT IS A CHEMOTHERAPY DIET?

A chemotherapy diet, often known as a chemo-friendly or cancer-fighting diet, is a nutritional regimen intended to help those undergoing chemotherapy. It focuses on supplying vital nutrients, controlling adverse effects, and boosting general health throughout cancer therapy. The purpose of a chemo diet is to improve the body's ability to resist the physical and emotional hardships of chemotherapy, boost the immune system, and aid in recovery.

Here are important characteristics and principles related with a chemotherapy diet.

Nutrient-Rich Foods

The chemo diet prioritizes nutrient-dense foods that include critical vitamins, minerals, antioxidants, and other therapeutic components. These nutrients are essential for maintaining the immune system and overall health.

Protein for Healing

Protein is crucial for tissue regeneration and healing, especially for those undergoing chemotherapy. Lean protein foods such as poultry, fish, tofu, beans, and lentils are frequently used to aid in the recuperation process.

Balanced Macronutrients

The diet balances macronutrients such as proteins, carbs, and healthy fats. This equilibrium promotes prolonged energy and supports a variety of body activities.

Emphasis on Hydration

Maintaining proper hydration is vital throughout chemotherapy. Proper hydration reduces nausea, maintains renal function, and aids in the clearance of toxins from the body.

Antioxidant-Rich Foods

Antioxidants destroy free radicals, which may contribute to cancer growth. Fruits, vegetables, and whole grains high in antioxidants are frequently used to enhance the body's natural defense mechanisms.

Fiber for Digestive Health

Examples include whole grains, fruits, and vegetables, promote digestive health. They can assist with constipation, which is a typical adverse effect of some chemotherapy drugs.

Mindful Eating

Pay attention to your body's hunger and fullness signs. This method can assist people in managing appetite changes and maintaining a good connection with food during therapy.

Individualized Meal Planning

Tailor chemo diets to individual needs, tastes, and tolerances. Consulting with a licensed dietitian or nutritionist might assist in developing a tailored plan.

Minimizing Irritants

Certain meals and beverages might worsen side effects like nausea and mouth sores. The chemo diet may include avoiding or reducing these irritants to improve comfort and nutritional intake.

Safe Food Handling

Chemotherapy can impair the immune system, rendering people more vulnerable to illnesses. As a result, adhering to proper food handling procedures, such as washing hands and thoroughly heating foods, is critical for lowering the risk of foodborne infections.

IMPORTANCE OF NUTRITION DURING CHEMOTHERAPY

Nutrition is extremely important in helping those who are receiving chemotherapy. Chemotherapy has a significant impact on the body, affecting healthy tissues and organs as well as cancer cells. Proper diet during this difficult period is critical for various reasons:

Maintaining Strength and Energy

Chemotherapy can cause fatigue, a typical side effect that reduces the energy levels of those receiving treatment. Adequate diet, which includes a variety of macronutrients such as proteins, carbs, and fats, aids in energy maintenance, allowing patients to deal with the physical demands of treatment and daily living.

Supporting the immune system

Chemotherapy can impair the immune system, leaving people more vulnerable to infections. Nutrient-rich diets, particularly those high in vitamins and minerals, aid in the healthy functioning of the immune system. A well-nourished body is better able to resist infections and boost its natural defensive mechanisms.

Enhancing Healing and Recovery

Cancer treatment may damage healthy cells and tissues. Tissue repair and regeneration require enough nutrition, particularly a protein-rich diet. Proper healing is critical for reducing treatment-related problems and promoting overall recovery.

Managing side effects

Chemotherapy frequently produces side symptoms such as nausea, vomiting, and appetite disturbances. A well-planned diet can help alleviate these negative effects. Consuming small, frequent meals, staying hydrated, and eating foods that are easy on the digestive system can all help to relieve nausea and enhance overall comfort.

Preventing malnutrition

Malnutrition is a common issue among those following chemotherapy. The treatment process may cause a decrease in appetite, taste alterations, and trouble swallowing. These causes might lead to decreased food consumption and nutritional deficits. A well-planned diet can help avoid malnutrition by delivering needed nutrients in a tasty and accessible form to the patient.

Addressing weight changes

Chemotherapy can cause weight variations, including loss and increase. Maintaining a healthy weight is essential for general well-being and can improve treatment outcomes. Individual needs and preferences can be considered when designing nutrition interventions to assist people achieve and maintain a healthy weight.

Improving quality of life

Good diet improves the quality of life for people undergoing chemotherapy. It can improve mood, energy levels, and ability to participate in regular activities. Feeling well-nourished promotes well-being and resilience during the trials of cancer treatment.

Personalized Nutrition Plan

Each individual's response to chemotherapy is distinct, and nutritional requirements may differ. Consulting with a certified dietitian or nutritionist enables the creation of personalized nutrition regimens based on individual tastes, tolerances, and treatment goals.

IMPORTANCE OF HYDRATION DURING TREATMENT

Hydration is essential for overall health, especially during cancer treatment, which includes chemotherapy. Proper fluid intake is critical for many physiological systems and can have a substantial impact on a patient's overall health. Here are some significant factors that emphasize the significance of hydration during treatment:

Counteracting Dehydration

Chemotherapy may produce nausea, vomiting, diarrhea, and increased urination. These conditions could lead to fluid loss and dehydration. Adequate hydration helps to counteract these effects and maintain the body's fluid balance.

Supporting Kidney Function

Adequate hydration is essential for kidney health, as some chemotherapy medications are removed through the kidneys. Staying hydrated allows the kidneys to eliminate toxins and metabolic wastes more efficiently.

Managing Nausea and Vomiting

Hydration can reduce nausea and vomiting, which are common side effects of chemotherapy. Drinking clear fluids, such as water or herbal teas, can help to relieve symptoms and prevent dehydration.

Preventing Constipation

Certain cancer therapies and drugs may cause constipation. Adequate fluid intake, combined with a fiber-rich diet, can help prevent and reduce this common side effect.

Improving Energy Levels

Dehydration can lead to weariness and weakness. Staying hydrated boosts energy levels, allowing patients to better handle the physical demands of cancer therapy.

Enhancing Nutrient Absorption:

Hydration promotes nutrient digestion and absorption. This is especially important for people receiving chemotherapy because good nutrition is essential for general health and recovery.

Minimizing Mouth and Throat Issues

Hydration can help with dry mouth and throat, which are common adverse effects of chemotherapy. Sipping water throughout the day and nibbling on ice chips can help.

Temperature Regulation

Maintaining sufficient hydration helps maintain body temperature, especially during fevers and treatment-related changes.

Promoting Skin Health

Hydration is crucial for preserving skin health. Cancer therapies, particularly radiation therapy, can have an effect on the skin, and staying hydrated can help lessen these effects.

KEY NUTRIENTS FOR CANCER PATIENTS

1. **Protein**

    - Essential for maintaining muscle mass.
    - Found in lean meats, poultry, fish, eggs, dairy products, legumes, and plant-based protein sources.

2. **Calories**

    - Adequate calorie intake is essential to prevent weight loss and support energy levels.
    - Focus on nutrient-dense foods to meet calorie needs.

3. **Carbohydrates**

    - Serve as a major source of fuel and supply energy.
    - Example include whole grains, fruits, and vegetables.

4. **Fats**

- They are essential for overall health.
- Example includes avocados, nuts, seeds, and olive oil.

5. **Vitamins**
   - Vitamin A, C, and E have antioxidant properties and support immune function.
   - There are gotten in fruits, vegetables, nuts, and seeds.

6. **Minerals**
   - Calcium and vitamin D for bone health.
   - Iron for preventing anemia.
   - Zinc and selenium for immune support.
   - They are gotten from dairy products, leafy greens, nuts, seeds, and lean meats.

7. **Fiber**
    - Important for digestive health.
    - Found in whole grains, fruits, vegetables, legumes, and nuts.

8. **Water**
    - It's important to stay properly hydrated, particularly if you're having adverse effects like nausea or diarrhea.
    - Take a lot of water, herbal teas, and clear broths.

9. **Omega-3 Fatty Acids**
    - Anti-inflammatory and may support overall health.
    - Found in walnuts, flaxseeds, chia seeds, and fatty fish (salmon, mackerel).

10. **Prebiotics and Probiotics**
    - Support gut health, which is important for overall well-being.

- Prebiotics are found in certain fruits and vegetables, while probiotics are found in fermented foods like yogurt and kefir.

11. **Antioxidants**

    - Found in a variety of fruits and vegetables, antioxidants help protect cells from damage.

BUILDING A BALANCED MEAL

Choosing the Right Proteins

During chemotherapy, integrating the correct proteins into your diet is critical for maintaining muscle mass and improving overall health. Choose lean protein sources that are easy to digest and include needed amino acids. Consider the following choices.

- **Lean Meats:** Skinless chicken, lean beef or pork chops.
- **Fish:** Fatty fish like salmon, mackerel, and trout for omega-3 fatty acids.
- **Plant-Based Proteins:** Tofu, beans, lentils, and chickpeas.
- **Dairy:** Low-fat or fat-free dairy products like yogurt and cottage cheese.
- **Eggs:** They are easily digestible source of protein.

Balancing protein intake throughout the day can help manage energy levels and support the body's healing process.

Incorporating Healthy Carbohydrates

Carbohydrates are an important source of energy and should be included in a well-balanced diet. Focus on complex carbs, which provide long-term energy and important elements. Consider including:

- **Whole Grains:** Brown rice, quinoa, oats, and whole wheat products.

- **Fruits:** Fresh or frozen fruits rich in vitamins, minerals, and fiber.

- **Vegetables:** Colorful and leafy vegetables to enhance nutritional variety.

- **Legumes:** Beans and lentils for a good source of fiber and protein.

Including Essential Fats

Healthy fats are necessary for food absorption, cognitive function, and overall health. To promote heart health, eat foods high in unsaturated fats and omega-3 fats. Add the following to your diet:

- **Avocados:** Rich in monounsaturated fats and a good source of vitamins.

- **Nuts and Seeds:** Almonds, walnuts, chia seeds, and flaxseeds for omega-3s.

- **Olive Oil:** Extra virgin olive oil should be used for cooking and salad dressings.

- **Fatty Fish:** Salmon, tuna, and sardines for omega-3 fatty acids.

COMBATING COMMON SIDE EFFECTS

Managing Nausea through Diet

Nausea is a typical side effect of chemotherapy, and following the proper dietary guidelines can help decrease discomfort. Consider the following tips:

- **Ginger:** Incorporate ginger into your diet through ginger tea, ginger candies, or adding it to meals. It has anti-nausea properties.

- **Small, Frequent Meals:** Opt for smaller, more frequent meals rather than large ones to avoid overwhelming your stomach.

- **Bland Foods:** Choose mild and easily digestible foods such as crackers, plain rice, and bananas.

- **Stay Hydrated:** Sip on clear liquids throughout the day to prevent dehydration. Try herbal teas, broth, or electrolyte-rich drinks.

Foods to Combat Fatigue

Fatigue is a common issue for those going through chemotherapy, but certain foods might provide a natural energy boost. Consider these fatigue-fighting options:

- **Complex Carbohydrates:** Vegetables, fruits, and whole grains offer long-lasting energy.

- **Lean Proteins:** Incorporate lean proteins like chicken, fish, and legumes for a protein boost without excessive fat.

- **Hydration:** Dehydration can contribute to fatigue, so ensure you're staying well-hydrated with water and other hydrating beverages.

- **Snack Smart:** Opt for nutrient-dense snacks like nuts, yogurt, or fresh fruit to keep your energy levels stable throughout the day.

Maintaining Appetite during Treatment

Chemotherapy can occasionally cause lack of appetite, making it difficult to meet nutritional needs. To maintain appetite and guarantee proper nutrient intake, consider the following suggestions:

- **Frequent, Small Meals:** Eat smaller meals more frequently throughout the day rather than three large meals.

- **Flavorful Foods:** Choose flavorful options using herbs, spices, and condiments to enhance the taste of your meals.

- **High-Calorie Snacks:** Snack on calorie-dense foods like nuts, cheese, and dried fruits to boost overall calorie intake.

- **Stay Hydrated:** Drink liquids between meals rather than with meals to avoid feeling too full.

FOOD TO EAT AND FOOD TO AVOID

Foods to Include

1. **Lean Proteins**
   - Chicken, turkey, fish, tofu, lentils, and eggs include needed amino acids for muscle maintenance.

2. **Whole Grains**
   - Brown rice, quinoa, oats, and whole wheat products provide fiber and sustained energy.

3. **Fruits and Vegetables**
   - Colored fruits and vegetables include vitamins, minerals, antioxidants, and fiber.

4. **Healthy Fats**
   - Avocados, nuts, seeds, and olive oil include healthy fats that promote general well-being.

5. **Hydration**
    - Stay hydrated with water, herbal teas, and clear broths, especially when experiencing nausea or diarrhea.

6. **Dairy or Dairy Alternatives**
    - Low-fat or fat-free choices contain calcium and vitamin D, which promote bone health.

7. **Ginger**
    - Ginger has anti-nausea effects and can be consumed in teas or meals.

8. **Soft, Moist Foods**
    - Soft and moist foods, such as cooked or steamed vegetables, soups, and stews, are easier to digest.

9. **Small, Frequent Meals**
    - Eating smaller, more frequent meals can help with nausea and energy levels.

10. **Probiotics**
    - Yogurt with active microorganisms can improve intestinal health.

Foods to Avoid or Limit

1. **Processed Foods**
    - Limit processed foods with high salt, sugar, and harmful fats.

2. **Sugary Snacks and Beverages**
    - Limit sugary snacks and drinks to maintain stable blood sugar levels.

3. **Spicy and Acidic Foods**
    - Some people may experience digestive difficulties or mouth irritation when eating these foods.

4. **Alcohol**
    - Limit or avoid alcohol, especially if it interferes with drugs or raises concerns about liver function.

5. **Raw or Undercooked Foods**
   - Avoid raw or undercooked foods to lessen illness risk.

6. **High-Fiber Foods**
   - Reducing fiber intake may help with digestive difficulties.

7. **Very Hot or Cold Foods**
   - Hot or cold foods might cause discomfort for those with sensitive mouths.

8. **Foods with Strong Odors**
   - Strong-smelling foods may be unpleasant for those experiencing taste or smell alterations.

CHAPTER 1

Breakfast recipes

1. Berry Protein Smoothie Bowl

Ingredients

- Mixed berries (strawberries, blueberries, raspberries) of 1 Cup
- 1 banana
- 1/2 cup Greek yogurt
- 1 scoop protein powder (whey or plant-based)
- 1 tablespoon honey
- 1/4 cup granola (optional for topping)

Preparation

1. Blend berries, banana, Greek yogurt, protein powder, and honey until smooth.
2. Pour into a bowl and top with granola if desired.

Nutritional Information

- Protein: 20g
- Fiber: 5g
- Calories: 300

Serving Size: 1 bowl

Preparation Time: 5 minutes

2. Oatmeal with Almond Butter and Banana Slices

Ingredients

- 1/2 cup rolled oats
- 1 cup almond milk
- 1 tablespoon almond butter
- 1 banana, sliced
- 1 teaspoon chia seeds (optional)

Preparation

1. Cook oats in almond milk until creamy.
2. Stir in almond butter and top with banana slices and chia seeds.

Nutritional Information

- Protein: 8g
- Fiber: 6g
- Calories: 300

Serving Size: 1 bowl

Preparation Time: 10 minutes

3. Avocado and Tomato Breakfast Toast

Ingredients

- 1 slice whole-grain bread
- 1/2 avocado, mashed
- Cherry tomatoes, sliced
- Sprinkle of salt and pepper
- Fresh basil leaves (optional)

Preparation

1. Toast the bread slice.
2. Spread mashed avocado on the toast and top with sliced tomatoes.

3. Season with salt, pepper, and garnish with fresh basil.

Nutritional Information

- Protein: 6g
- Fiber: 8g
- Calories: 250

Serving Size: 1 slice

Preparation Time: 5 minutes

4. Coconut and Mango Chia Pudding

Ingredients

- 2 tablespoons chia seeds
- 1/2 cup coconut milk
- 1/2 cup diced mango
- 1 tablespoon shredded coconut (unsweetened)

Preparation

1. Mix chia seeds and coconut milk, let it sit in the refrigerator for a few hours or overnight.

2. Layer chia pudding with diced mango and shredded coconut.

Nutritional Information

- Protein: 7g
- Fiber: 10g
- Calories: 280

Serving Size: 1 jar

Preparation Time: 5 minutes (plus chilling time)

5. Spinach and Feta Egg Muffins
Ingredients

- 4 eggs
- 1 cup fresh spinach, chopped
- 1/4 cup feta cheese, crumbled
- Salt and pepper to taste

Preparation

1. Preheat the oven to 350°F (175°C).
2. Whisk eggs and mix in chopped spinach, feta, salt, and pepper.
3. Pour the mixture into greased muffin cups and bake for 15-20 minutes.

Nutritional Information

- Protein: 15g
- Fiber: 2g
- Calories: 220

Serving Size: 2 muffins

Preparation Time: 20 minutes

6. Banana Walnut Breakfast Cookies

Ingredients

- 2 ripe bananas, mashed
- 1 cup rolled oats
- 1/4 cup chopped walnuts
- 1 tablespoon honey
- 1/2 teaspoon cinnamon

Preparation

1. Preheat the oven to 350°F (175°C).
2. Mix mashed bananas, oats, walnuts, honey, and cinnamon.
3. Drop spoonfuls onto a baking sheet and bake for 12-15 minutes.

Nutritional Information

- Protein: 5g
- Fiber: 4g
- Calories: 180

Serving Size: 2 cookies

Preparation Time: 15 minutes

7. Quinoa Breakfast Bowl
Ingredients

- 1/2 cup cooked quinoa
- 1/2 cup almond milk
- 1 tablespoon honey
- Fresh berries
- Sliced almonds

Preparation

1. Mix cooked quinoa with almond milk and drizzle honey.
2. Top with fresh berries and sliced almonds.

Nutritional Information

- Protein: 8g
- Fiber: 5g
- Calories: 270

- **Serving Size**: 1 bowl
- **Preparation Time**: 10 minutes

8. Cottage Cheese and Pineapple Parfait

Ingredients

- 1/2 cup low-fat cottage cheese
- 1/2 cup diced pineapple
- 1 tablespoon flaxseeds (ground)

Preparation

1. Layer cottage cheese with diced pineapple in a glass.
2. Sprinkle ground flaxseeds on top.

Nutritional Information

- Protein: 15g
- Fiber: 3g
- Calories: 220

Serving Size: 1 parfait

Preparation Time: 5 minutes

9. Sweet Potato and Spinach Frittata

Ingredients

- 2 eggs
- 1/2 cup cooked sweet potatoes, diced
- Handful of fresh spinach, chopped
- Salt and pepper to taste

Preparation

1. Preheat the oven to 350°F (175°C).
2. Whisk eggs and mix in sweet potatoes, spinach, salt, and pepper.
3. Pour the mixture into a greased oven-safe pan and bake for 15-20 minutes.

Nutritional Information

- Protein: 12g
- Fiber: 3g
- Calories: 230

Serving Size: 1/4 frittata

Preparation Time: 20 minutes

10. Blueberry Almond Chia Seed Pudding

Ingredients

- 3 tablespoons chia seeds
- 1 cup almond milk
- 1/2 cup blueberries
- 1 tablespoon almond slices

Preparation

1. Mix chia seeds and almond milk, let it sit in the refrigerator for a few hours or overnight.
2. Layer chia pudding with blueberries and almond slices.

Nutritional Information

- Protein: 7g
- Fiber: 9g
- Calories: 280

Serving Size: 1 jar

Preparation Time: 5 minutes (plus chilling time)

11. Peanut Butter Banana Toast

Ingredients

- 1 slice whole-grain bread
- 2 tablespoons peanut butter
- 1 banana, sliced
- Drizzle of honey (optional)

Preparation

1. Toast the bread slice.
2. Spread peanut butter on the toast and top with banana slices.
3. Drizzle with honey if desired.

Nutritional Information

- Protein: 8g
- Fiber: 6g
- Calories: 320

Serving Size: 1 slice

Preparation Time: 5 minutes

12. Yogurt and Granola Parfait

Ingredients

- 1/2 cup Greek yogurt
- 1/4 cup granola
- 1/2 cup mixed berries (strawberries, blueberries)

Preparation

1. Layer Greek yogurt with granola in a glass.
2. Top with mixed berries.

Nutritional Information

- Protein: 15g
- Fiber: 4g
- Calories: 250

Serving Size: 1 parfait

Preparation Time: 5 minutes

13. Apple Cinnamon Overnight Oats

Ingredients

- 1/2 cup rolled oats
- 1/2 cup almond milk
- 1/2 apple, grated
- 1/2 teaspoon cinnamon

Preparation

1. Mix oats, almond milk, grated apple, and cinnamon in a jar.
2. Let it sit in the refrigerator overnight.
3. Stir before serving.

Nutritional Information

- Protein: 7g
- Fiber: 6g
- Calories: 230

Serving Size: 1 jar

Preparation Time: 5 minutes (plus chilling time)

14. Mango Coconut Rice Pudding

Ingredients

- 1/2 cup cooked brown rice
- 1/2 cup coconut milk
- 1/2 cup diced mango
- 1 tablespoon shredded coconut (unsweetened)

Preparation

1. Mix cooked brown rice with coconut milk and diced mango.
2. Top with shredded coconut.

Nutritional Information

- Protein: 5g
- Fiber: 4g
- Calories: 270

Serving Size: 1 bowl

Preparation Time: 10 minutes

CHAPTER 2

Lunch Recipes

1. Chicken and Quinoa Bowl

Ingredients

- Cooked chicken breast
- Quinoa
- Steamed broccoli
- Carrots, julienned
- Olive oil
- Lemon juice
- Fresh parsley
- Salt, pepper

Preparation

- Mix cooked quinoa with shredded chicken, steamed broccoli, and julienned carrots.
- Dress with olive oil, lemon juice, and season with salt and pepper.
- Garnish with fresh parsley.

Nutritional Information

- Calories: 350
- Protein: 25g
- Carbohydrates: 30g
- Dietary Fiber: 6g

Serving Size: 1 bowl

Preparation Time: 25 minutes

2. Salmon and Quinoa Salad

Ingredients

- Grilled salmon fillet
- Quinoa
- Mixed greens
- Cherry tomatoes, halved
- Cucumber, sliced
- Balsamic vinaigrette
- Lemon zest
- Salt, pepper

Preparation

- Combine cooked quinoa, mixed greens, cherry tomatoes, and cucumber. Top with grilled salmon.
- Drizzle with balsamic vinaigrette, sprinkle lemon zest.
- Season with salt and pepper.

Nutritional Information

- Calories: 400
- Protein: 30g
- Carbohydrates: 35g
- Dietary Fiber: 7g

Serving Size: 1 salad

Preparation Time: 30 minutes

3. Vegetarian Quinoa Stir-Fry

Ingredients

- Quinoa
- Tofu, cubed
- Broccoli florets
- Bell peppers, sliced
- Snow peas
- Soy sauce (low-sodium)
- Sesame oil
- Ginger, minced
- Garlic, minced

Preparation

- Cook quinoa. In a pan, stir-fry tofu, broccoli, bell peppers, and snow peas in sesame oil.
- Add soy sauce, ginger, and garlic.
- Mix with cooked quinoa.

Nutritional Information

- Calories: 320
- Protein: 20g
- Carbohydrates: 40g
- Dietary Fiber: 8g

Serving Size: 1.5 cups

Preparation Time: 25 minutes

4. Mango Avocado Chickpea Salad

Ingredients

- Chickpeas, canned
- Mango, diced
- Avocado, diced
- Red onion, finely chopped
- Cilantro, chopped
- Lime juice
- Olive oil
- Salt, pepper

Preparation

- Rinse and drain chickpeas.
- Combine with mango, avocado, red onion, and cilantro. Dress with lime juice, olive oil.
- Season with salt and pepper.

Nutritional Information

- Calories: 280
- Protein: 9g
- Carbohydrates: 40g
- Dietary Fiber: 10g

Serving Size: 1.5 cups

Preparation Time: 20 minutes

5. Turkey and Vegetable Skewers

Ingredients

- Turkey breast, cubed
- Zucchini, sliced
- Cherry tomatoes
- Bell peppers, diced
- Olive oil
- Lemon juice
- Oregano, dried
- Garlic powder
- Salt, pepper

Preparation

- Thread turkey, zucchini, cherry tomatoes, and bell peppers onto skewers.
- Brush with a mixture of olive oil, lemon juice, dried oregano, garlic powder, salt, and pepper.
- Grill until cooked.

Nutritional Information

- Calories: 290
- Protein: 30g
- Carbohydrates: 15g
- Dietary Fiber: 5g

Serving Size: 2 skewers

Preparation Time: 30 minutes

6. Lemon Garlic Shrimp Pasta
Ingredients

- Whole wheat pasta
- Shrimp, peeled and deveined
- Broccoli florets
- Garlic, minced
- Lemon zest
- Olive oil
- Parsley, chopped
- Salt, pepper

Preparation

- Cook pasta. Sauté shrimp, broccoli, and minced garlic in olive oil.
- Toss with cooked pasta.
- Garnish with lemon zest and parsley.
- Season with salt and pepper.

Nutritional Information

- Calories: 350
- Protein: 25g
- Carbohydrates: 45g
- Dietary Fiber: 8g

Serving Size: 1.5 cups

Preparation Time: 25 minutes

7. Spinach and Feta Stuffed Chicken Breast

Ingredients

- Chicken breast, boneless
- Spinach, chopped
- Feta cheese, crumbled
- Garlic, minced
- Olive oil
- Lemon juice
- Paprika
- Salt, pepper

Preparation

- Preheat oven.
- Mix chopped spinach, crumbled feta, minced garlic, olive oil, and lemon juice.
- Cut a pocket in the chicken breast, stuff with the spinach mixture. Season with paprika, salt, and pepper.
- Bake until cooked.

Nutritional Information

- Calories: 320
- Protein: 35g
- Carbohydrates: 5g
- Dietary Fiber: 2g

Serving Size: 1 stuffed breast

Preparation Time: 35 minutes

8. Cauliflower and Broccoli Soup

Ingredients

- Cauliflower, chopped
- Broccoli, chopped
- Onion, diced
- Garlic, minced
- Vegetable broth (low-sodium)
- Greek yogurt
- Nutmeg, ground
- Salt, pepper

Preparation

- Sauté onion and garlic.
- Add cauliflower, broccoli, and vegetable broth.
- Simmer until vegetables are tender.
- Blend with Greek yogurt, ground nutmeg, salt, and pepper.

Nutritional Information

- Calories: 150
- Protein: 8g
- Carbohydrates: 20g
- Dietary Fiber: 6g

Serving Size: 1.5 cups

Preparation Time: 30 minutes

9. Egg and Vegetable Wrap

Ingredients

- Eggs, beaten
- Whole wheat wrap
- Spinach, chopped
- Bell peppers, diced
- Tomato, sliced
- Avocado, sliced
- Salsa
- Salt, pepper

Preparation

- Scramble eggs.
- Fill a whole wheat wrap with scrambled eggs, chopped spinach, diced bell peppers, tomato slices, avocado slices, and salsa.
- Season with salt and pepper.

Nutritional Information

- Calories: 320
- Protein: 15g
- Carbohydrates: 25g
- Dietary Fiber: 7g

Serving Size: 1 wrap

Preparation Time: 15 minutes

10. Sweet Potato and Black Bean Chili

Ingredients

- Sweet potatoes, diced
- Black beans, canned
- Onion, diced
- Garlic, minced
- Vegetable broth (low-sodium)
- Tomatoes, diced
- Chili powder
- Cumin, ground

- Paprika
- Salt, pepper

Preparation

- Sauté onion and garlic.
- Add sweet potatoes, black beans, vegetable broth, diced tomatoes, chili powder, ground cumin, paprika, salt, and pepper.
- Simmer until sweet potatoes are cooked.

Nutritional Information

- Calories: 280
- Protein: 10g
- Carbohydrates: 55g
- Dietary Fiber: 14g

Serving Size: 1.5 cups

Preparation Time: 35 minutes

CHAPTER 3

Dinner Recipes

1. Salmon and Sweet Potato Skewers

Ingredients

- Salmon fillets
- Sweet potatoes, cubed
- Olive oil
- Lemon
- Fresh dill
- Salt, pepper

Preparation

- Salmon should be marinated in olive oil, lemon juice, and dill.
- Thread onto skewers with cubed sweet potatoes.
- Grill until salmon is cooked through.

Nutritional Information

- Calories: 350
- Protein: 25g
- Carbohydrates: 20g
- Dietary Fiber: 3g

Serving Size: 1 skewer

Preparation Time: 30 minutes

2. Baked Lemon Garlic Chicken

Ingredients

- Chicken thighs
- Lemon
- Garlic, minced
- Olive oil
- Thyme
- Rosemary
- Salt, pepper

Preparation

- Marinate chicken in a mixture of lemon, garlic, olive oil, thyme, rosemary, salt, and pepper.
- Bake until golden.

Nutritional Information

- Calories: 280
- Protein: 30g
- Carbohydrates: 2g
- Dietary Fiber: 0g

Serving Size: 2 thighs

Preparation Time: 40 minutes

3. Chickpea and Spinach Curry

Ingredients

- Chickpeas, canned
- Spinach
- Coconut milk
- Onion, diced
- Tomatoes, diced
- Ginger, minced
- Garlic, minced
- Curry powder
- Turmeric
- Cumin
- Coriander
- Olive oil
- Salt, pepper

Preparation

- Onions, ginger, and garlic should be saunted in olive oil.
- Add chickpeas, tomatoes, and spices.
- Stir in coconut milk and spinach.
- Simmer until spinach wilts.

Nutritional Information

- Calories: 320
- Protein: 15g
- Carbohydrates: 30g
- Dietary Fiber: 10g

Serving Size: 1.5 cups

Preparation Time: 30 minutes

4. Turkey and Vegetable Skillet

Ingredients

- Ground turkey
- Zucchini, diced
- Bell peppers, sliced
- Onion, diced
- Tomato sauce
- Italian seasoning
- Olive oil
- Salt, pepper

Preparation

- Sauté ground turkey in olive oil.
- Add vegetables, tomato sauce, and Italian seasoning. Simmer until vegetables are tender.

Nutritional Information

- Calories: 290
- Protein: 20g

- Carbohydrates: 15g
- Dietary Fiber: 4g

Serving Size: 1 cup

Preparation Time: 25 minutes

5. Mushroom and Brown Rice Risotto
Ingredients

- Brown rice
- Mushrooms, sliced
- Onion, diced
- Garlic, minced
- Vegetable broth
- Parmesan cheese
- White wine (optional)
- Olive oil
- Salt, pepper

Preparation

- Onion and garlic should be Sautéd in olive oil.
- Add mushrooms, rice, and white wine.
- Gradually add vegetable broth, stirring until rice is cooked. Finish with Parmesan.

Nutritional Information

- Calories: 280
- Protein: 8g
- Carbohydrates: 40g
- Dietary Fiber: 5g
- Iron: 15%

Serving Size: 1 cup

Preparation Time: 35 minutes

6. Lemon Herb Baked Cod

Ingredients

- Cod fillets
- Lemon
- Fresh parsley, chopped
- Dill, chopped
- Garlic, minced
- Olive oil
- Salt, pepper

Preparation

- Marinate cod in a mixture of lemon, garlic, olive oil, parsley, dill, salt, and pepper.
- Bake until fish flakes easily.

Nutritional Information

- Calories: 250
- Protein: 25g

- Carbohydrates: 1g
- Dietary Fiber: 0g

Serving Size: 1 fillet

Preparation Time: 25 minutes

7. Vegetable and Lentil Soup

Ingredients

- Green lentils
- Carrots, diced
- Celery, diced
- Onion, diced
- Garlic, minced
- Vegetable broth
- Tomatoes, diced
- Thyme, bay leaves
- Olive oil
- Salt, pepper

Preparation

- Sauté onion, garlic, carrots, and celery in olive oil.
- Add lentils, tomatoes, thyme, bay leaves, and vegetable broth.
- Simmer until lentils are tender.

Nutritional Information

- Calories: 220
- Protein: 12g
- Carbohydrates: 35g
- Dietary Fiber: 10g

Serving Size: 1.5 cups

Preparation Time: 40 minutes

8. Shrimp and Broccoli Stir-Fry

Ingredients

- Shrimp
- Broccoli florets
- Carrots, julienned
- Soy sauce
- Ginger, minced
- Garlic, minced
- Olive oil
- Brown rice

Preparation

- Stir-fry shrimp, broccoli, and carrots in olive oil with ginger and garlic.
- Add soy sauce.
- Serve over cooked brown rice.

Nutritional Information

- Calories: 300
- Protein: 25g
- Carbohydrates: 30g
- Dietary Fiber: 5g

CHAPTER 4

Appetizers and snacks

1. Hummus and Veggie Platter

Ingredients

- Chickpeas
- Tahini
- Lemon juice
- Garlic
- Olive oil
- Salt
- Assorted vegetables for dipping (carrots, cucumber, bell peppers)

Preparation

1. Blend chickpeas, tahini, lemon juice, garlic, olive oil, and salt until smooth.
2. Serve with sliced vegetables.

Nutritional Information

- Calories: 150
- Protein: 5g
- Carbohydrates: 20g
- Dietary Fiber: 5g

Serving Size: Approximately 1/2 cup of hummus with a serving of assorted vegetables.

Preparation Time: 10 minutes

2. Greek Yogurt and Berry Parfait

Ingredients

- Greek yogurt
- Mixed berries (strawberries, blueberries, raspberries)
- Honey
- Granola

Preparation

1. Layer Greek yogurt with mixed berries and granola.

2. Drizzle honey on top.

Nutritional Information

- Calories: 200
- Protein: 15g
- Carbohydrates: 30g
- Dietary Fiber: 5g

Serving Size: 1 cup of parfait.

Preparation Time: 5 minutes

3. Avocado and Tomato Salsa with Whole Grain Chips
Ingredients

- Avocado
- Tomatoes
- Red onion
- Cilantro
- Lime juice
- Salt
- Whole grain tortilla chips

Preparation

1. Dice avocado, tomatoes, and red onion.
2. Mix with chopped cilantro, lime juice, and salt.
3. Serve with whole grain tortilla chips.

Nutritional Information

- Calories: 180
- Protein: 3g
- Carbohydrates: 20g
- Dietary Fiber: 6g

Serving Size: Approximately 1/2 cup of salsa with a serving of whole grain tortilla chips.

Preparation Time: 15 minutes

4. Cucumber and Smoked Salmon Rolls

Ingredients

- Cucumber
- Smoked salmon
- Cream cheese
- Dill

Preparation

1. Slice cucumber lengthwise into thin strips.
2. Spread cream cheese on each strip, add a piece of smoked salmon, and roll.
3. Garnish with dill.

Nutritional Information

- Calories: 120
- Protein: 12g
- Carbohydrates: 2g
- Dietary Fiber: 0g

Serving Size: Approximately 4 rolls.

Preparation Time: 10 minutes

5. Edamame and Sea Salt
Ingredients

- Edamame (soybeans)
- Sea salt

Preparation

1. Boil or steam edamame until tender.
2. Sprinkle with sea salt.

Nutritional Information

- Calories: 120
- Protein: 13g
- Carbohydrates: 9g
- Dietary Fiber: 5g

Serving Size: Approximately 1 cup.

Preparation Time: 10 minutes

6. Caprese Skewers

Ingredients

- Cherry tomatoes
- Fresh mozzarella balls
- Basil leaves
- Balsamic glaze

Preparation

1. Put basil leaves, mozzarella balls, and cherry tomatoes on skewers.
2. Drizzle with balsamic glaze.

Nutritional Information

- Calories: 160
- Protein: 10g
- Carbohydrates: 5g
- Dietary Fiber: 1g

Serving Size: Approximately 3 skewers.

Preparation Time: 15 minutes

7. Roasted Red Pepper and White Bean Dip

Ingredients

- Roasted red peppers
- Cannellini beans
- Garlic
- Lemon juice
- Olive oil
- Cumin
- Paprika
- Salt

Preparation

1. Blend roasted red peppers, cannellini beans, garlic, lemon juice, olive oil, cumin, paprika, and salt until smooth.
2. Serve with whole grain crackers.

Nutritional Information

- Calories: 140
- Protein: 4g
- Carbohydrates: 18g
- Dietary Fiber: 4g

Serving Size: Approximately 1/4 cup of dip with a serving of whole grain crackers.

Preparation Time: 10 minutes

8. Baked Sweet Potato Fries

Ingredients

- Sweet potatoes
- Olive oil
- Paprika
- Garlic powder
- Salt

Preparation

1. Cut sweet potatoes into fries, toss with olive oil, paprika, garlic powder, and salt.

2. Bake until crispy.

Nutritional Information

- Calories: 120
- Protein: 2g
- Carbohydrates: 26g
- Dietary Fiber: 4g

Serving Size: Approximately 1 cup of fries.

Preparation Time: 25 minutes

9. Turkey and Cranberry Lettuce Wraps

Ingredients

- Turkey slices
- Cranberry sauce
- Lettuce leaves

Preparation

1. Lay turkey slices on lettuce leaves.

2. Add a dollop of cranberry sauce and roll into wraps.

Nutritional Information

- Calories: 90
- Protein: 15g
- Carbohydrates: 5g
- Dietary Fiber: 1g

Serving Size: 2 wraps.

Preparation Time: 10 minutes

CHAPTER 5

Soup and Stews Recipes

1. Healing Chicken and Rice Soup

Ingredients

- Cooked chicken breast
- Brown rice
- Carrots
- Celery
- Low-sodium chicken broth
- Onion
- Garlic
- Thyme, bay leaves, salt, pepper

Preparation

- Sauté onion and garlic, add carrots, celery, cooked chicken, brown rice, and chicken broth.
- Simmer with thyme and bay leaves.

Nutritional Information

- Calories: 250
- Protein: 20g
- Carbohydrates: 30g
- Dietary Fiber: 4g
- Sugars: 2g

Serving Size: 1.5 cups

Preparation Time: 35 minutes

2. Vegetarian Lentil and Spinach Stew

Ingredients

- Green lentils
- Spinach
- Carrots
- Onion
- Garlic
- Vegetable broth
- Tomatoes
- Cumin, coriander, turmeric, salt, pepper

Preparation

- Sauté onion and garlic, add lentils, spinach, carrots, tomatoes, and spices.
- Pour in vegetable broth and simmer until lentils are tender.

Nutritional Information

- Calories: 220
- Protein: 15g
- Carbohydrates: 35g
- Dietary Fiber: 10g

Serving Size: 1.5 cups

Preparation Time: 40 minutes

3. Creamy Butternut Squash Soup
Ingredients

- Butternut squash
- Onion
- Garlic
- Low-sodium vegetable broth
- Coconut milk
- Nutmeg, cinnamon, salt, pepper

Preparation

- Roast butternut squash, sauté onion and garlic, blend with vegetable broth, coconut milk, and spices until smooth.

Nutritional Information

- Calories: 180
- Protein: 2g
- Carbohydrates: 30g
- Dietary Fiber: 5g

Serving Size: 1 cup

Preparation Time: 45 minutes

4. Salmon and Vegetable Chowder

Ingredients

- Salmon fillet
- Potatoes
- Carrots
- Celery
- Onion
- Low-sodium chicken broth
- Milk
- Dill, salt, pepper

Preparation

- Sauté onion, add potatoes, carrots, celery, chicken broth, and milk.
- Simmer until vegetables are tender, then add flaked salmon and dill.

Nutritional Information

- Calories: 280
- Protein: 25g
- Carbohydrates: 25g
- Dietary Fiber: 4g

Serving Size: 1.5 cups

Preparation Time: 35 minutes

5. Tomato Basil and Chickpea Stew

Ingredients

- Canned chickpeas
- Tomatoes
- Onion
- Garlic
- Low-sodium vegetable broth
- Fresh basil
- Olive oil, salt, pepper

Preparation

- Sauté onion and garlic, add chickpeas, tomatoes, vegetable broth, and fresh basil.
- Simmer until flavors meld.

Nutritional Information

- Calories: 210
- Protein: 8g
- Carbohydrates: 35g
- Dietary Fiber: 8g

Serving Size: 1.5 cups

Preparation Time: 30 minutes

6. Chicken and Vegetable Noodle Soup

Ingredients

- Cooked chicken breast
- Whole wheat noodles
- Carrots
- Celery
- Low-sodium chicken broth
- Onion
- Garlic
- Thyme, bay leaves, salt, pepper

Preparation

- Sauté onion and garlic, add carrots, celery, cooked chicken, whole wheat noodles, and chicken broth.
- Simmer with thyme and bay leaves.

Nutritional Information

- Calories: 270
- Protein: 20g

- Carbohydrates: 35g
- Dietary Fiber: 5g

Serving Size: 1.5 cups

Preparation Time: 40 minutes

7. Creamy Broccoli and Cauliflower Soup
Ingredients

- Broccoli
- Cauliflower
- Onion
- Garlic
- Low-sodium vegetable broth
- Greek yogurt
- Nutmeg, salt, pepper

Preparation

- Sauté onion and garlic, add broccoli, cauliflower, vegetable broth, and cook until vegetables are tender.

- Blend with Greek yogurt, nutmeg, salt, and pepper.

Nutritional Information

- Calories: 160
- Protein: 8g
- Carbohydrates: 25g
- Dietary Fiber: 8g

Serving Size: 1 cup

Preparation Time: 35 minutes

8. Spiced Lentil and Carrot Soup

Ingredients

- Red lentils
- Carrots
- Onion
- Garlic
- Low-sodium vegetable broth
- Cumin, coriander, turmeric, cinnamon, salt, pepper

Preparation

- Sauté onion and garlic, add red lentils, carrots, vegetable broth, and spices.
- Simmer until lentils are cooked and flavors meld.

Nutritional Information

- Calories: 230
- Protein: 12g
- Carbohydrates: 35g
- Dietary Fiber: 12g

Serving Size: 1.5 cups

Preparation Time: 40 minutes

9. Mushroom and Brown Rice Congee

Ingredients

- Brown rice
- Mushrooms
- Ginger
- Garlic
- Low-sodium vegetable broth
- Green onions
- Soy sauce, sesame oil, salt, pepper

Preparation

- Cook brown rice with vegetable broth until it breaks down into a porridge. Sauté mushrooms, ginger, and garlic separately.
- Combine, season with soy sauce, sesame oil, salt, and pepper.
- Top with green onions.

Nutritional Information

- Calories: 200
- Protein: 8g
- Carbohydrates: 40g
- Dietary Fiber: 5g

Serving Size: 1.5 cups

Preparation Time: 50 minutes

CHAPTER 6

Main Dish- Poultry Recipes

1. Lemon Herb Baked Chicken

Ingredients

- Chicken breast
- Lemon
- Garlic
- Fresh herbs (rosemary, thyme)
- Olive oil
- Salt, pepper

Preparation

- Marinate chicken in a mixture of lemon juice, minced garlic, chopped herbs, olive oil, salt, and pepper.
- Bake until fully cooked.

Nutritional Information

- Calories: 250
- Protein: 30g
- Carbohydrates: 2g
- Fat: 14g
- Fiber: 1g

Preparation Time: 30 minutes

Serving Size: 1 chicken breast (150g)

2. Turkey and Vegetable Stir-Fry

Ingredients

- Ground turkey
- Broccoli
- Bell peppers
- Snap peas
- Soy sauce (low-sodium)
- Garlic
- Ginger

- Olive oil

Preparation

- Brown ground turkey in olive oil, add vegetables, garlic, and ginger.
- Stir in soy sauce until vegetables are tender.

Nutritional Information

- Calories: 300
- Protein: 25g
- Carbohydrates: 10g
- Fat: 15g
- Fiber: 3g

Preparation Time: 25 minutes

Serving Size: 1 cup

3. Baked Pesto Chicken

Ingredients

- Chicken thighs
- Pesto sauce
- Cherry tomatoes
- Parmesan cheese

Preparation

- Coat chicken thighs with pesto sauce, top with halved cherry tomatoes and Parmesan cheese.
- Bake until chicken is cooked through.

Nutritional Information

- Calories: 280
- Protein: 22g
- Carbohydrates: 3g
- Fat: 20g
- Fiber: 1g

Preparation Time: 35 minutes

Serving Size: 2 thighs

4. Honey Mustard Grilled Chicken

Ingredients

- Chicken drumsticks
- Dijon mustard
- Honey
- Garlic
- Olive oil

Preparation

- Mix mustard, honey, minced garlic, and olive oil.
- Coat chicken drumsticks with the mixture and grill until fully cooked.

Nutritional Information

- Calories: 180
- Protein: 18g
- Carbohydrates: 10g
- Fat: 8g
- Fiber: 0.5g

Preparation Time: 30 minutes

Serving Size: 2 drumsticks

5. Herb Roasted Turkey Breast

Ingredients

- Turkey breast
- Fresh herbs (sage, thyme, rosemary)
- Garlic
- Lemon
- Olive oil

Preparation

- Rub turkey breast with minced garlic, chopped herbs, lemon zest, and olive oil.
- Roast until internal temperature reaches 165°F.

Nutritional Information

- Calories: 200
- Protein: 30g
- Carbohydrates: 1g

- Fat: 8g
- Fiber: 0.5g

Preparation Time: 40 minutes

Serving Size: 4 oz

6. Lemon Garlic Turkey Burgers
Ingredients

- Ground turkey
- Lemon
- Garlic
- Onion
- Whole wheat buns
- Lettuce, tomato (for toppings)

Preparation

- Mix ground turkey with minced garlic, grated onion, and lemon zest.
- Form into patties and grill.
- Serve on whole wheat buns with lettuce and tomato.

Nutritional Information

- Calories: 250
- Protein: 20g
- Carbohydrates: 25g
- Fat: 10g
- Fiber: 3g

Preparation Time: 25 minutes

Serving Size: 1 burger

7. Chicken and Brown Rice Casserole

Ingredients

- Chicken thighs
- Brown rice
- Carrots
- Peas
- Chicken broth
- Onion
- Garlic

- Herbs (thyme, parsley)

Preparation

- Sauté onion and garlic, add brown rice, chicken broth, vegetables, and chicken thighs.
- Bake until rice is tender.

Nutritional Information

- Calories: 300
- Protein: 22g
- Carbohydrates: 30g
- Fat: 10g
- Fiber: 4g

Preparation Time: 50 minutes

Serving Size: 1 cup

8. Orange Glazed Chicken

Ingredients

- Chicken drumsticks
- Orange juice
- Soy sauce (low-sodium)
- Honey
- Ginger
- Garlic

Preparation

- Mix orange juice, soy sauce, honey, minced ginger, and garlic.
- Coat chicken drumsticks with the mixture and bake until fully cooked.

Nutritional Information

- Calories: 220
- Protein: 18g
- Carbohydrates: 15g

- Fat: 10g
- Fiber: 0.5g

Preparation Time: 35 minutes

Serving Size: 2 drumsticks

9. Mango Salsa Turkey Tacos

Ingredients

- Ground turkey
- Whole wheat tortillas
- Mango
- Red onion
- Cilantro
- Lime
- Cumin, chili powder, salt

Preparation

- Brown ground turkey with cumin, chili powder, and salt.

- Make a salsa with diced mango, red onion, cilantro, and lime juice.
- Serve in whole wheat tortillas.

Nutritional Information

- Calories: 260
- Protein: 20g
- Carbohydrates: 30g
- Fat: 8g
- Fiber: 5g

Preparation Time: 30 minutes

Serving Size: 2 tacos

CHAPTER 7

Main Dish- Seafood Recipes

1. Baked Lemon Garlic Salmon

Ingredients

- Salmon fillets
- Lemon
- Garlic
- Olive oil
- Fresh dill
- Salt, pepper

Preparation

- Marinate salmon with lemon, garlic, olive oil, dill, salt, and pepper.
- Bake until cooked through.

Nutritional Information

- Calories: 300
- Protein: 25g
- Carbohydrates: 2g
- Fat: 20g
- Omega-3 Fatty Acids: 1,500mg

Serving Size: 1 fillet

Preparation Time: 20 minutes

2. Shrimp and Avocado Salad

Ingredients

- Shrimp
- Avocado
- Cherry tomatoes
- Red onion
- Cilantro
- Lime juice
- Olive oil

- Salt, pepper

Preparation

- Cook shrimp and toss with diced avocado, cherry tomatoes, red onion, cilantro, lime juice, olive oil, salt, and pepper.

Nutritional Information

- Calories: 250
- Protein: 20g
- Carbohydrates: 10g
- Fat: 15g
- Fiber: 5g

Serving Size: 1 cup

Preparation Time: 15 minutes

3. Grilled Lemon Herb Swordfish

Ingredients

- Swordfish steaks
- Lemon
- Fresh herbs (rosemary, thyme)
- Olive oil
- Garlic
- Salt, pepper

Preparation

- Marinate swordfish with lemon, fresh herbs, olive oil, garlic, salt, and pepper.
- Grill until fully cooked.

Nutritional Information

- Calories: 280
- Protein: 30g
- Carbohydrates: 2g
- Fat: 18g

- Omega-3 Fatty Acids: 900mg

Serving Size: 1 steak

Preparation Time: 25 minutes

4. Baked Cod with Tomato Salsa
Ingredients

- Cod fillets
- Tomatoes
- Red onion
- Cilantro
- Lime juice
- Olive oil
- Garlic
- Salt, pepper

Preparation

- Top cod fillets with a mixture of diced tomatoes, red onion, cilantro, lime juice, olive oil, garlic, salt, and pepper.

- Bake until fish flakes easily.

Nutritional Information

- Calories: 220
- Protein: 25g
- Carbohydrates: 8g
- Fat: 10g
- Fiber: 2g

Serving Size: 1 fillet

Preparation Time: 30 minutes

5. Lemon Garlic Butter Shrimp Pasta
Ingredients

- Shrimp
- Whole wheat pasta
- Lemon
- Garlic
- Butter
- Parsley

- Salt, pepper

Preparation

- Cook shrimp and toss with whole wheat pasta, lemon, garlic, butter, parsley, salt, and pepper.

Nutritional Information

- Calories: 350
- Protein: 25g
- Carbohydrates: 40g
- Fat: 12g
- Fiber: 6g

Serving Size: 1 cup

Preparation Time: 25 minutes

6. Teriyaki Glazed Salmon

Ingredients

- Salmon fillets
- Teriyaki sauce
- Honey
- Garlic
- Ginger
- Green onions
- Sesame seeds

Preparation

- Marinate salmon with a mixture of teriyaki sauce, honey, garlic, ginger, green onions, and sesame seeds.
- Bake until fully cooked.

Nutritional Information

- Calories: 280
- Protein: 30g
- Carbohydrates: 15g
- Fat: 10g
- **Serving Size**: 1 fillet
- **Preparation Time**: 30 minutes

7. Mango Salsa Tuna Salad

Ingredients

- Canned tuna
- Mango
- Red bell pepper
- Red onion
- Cilantro
- Lime juice
- Olive oil
- Salt, pepper

Preparation

- Combine canned tuna with diced mango, red bell pepper, red onion, cilantro, lime juice, olive oil, salt, and pepper.

Nutritional Information

- Calories: 230
- Protein: 25g
- Carbohydrates: 15g
- Fat: 10g
- Fiber: 2g

Serving Size: 1 cup

Preparation Time: 20 minutes

8. Cajun Grilled Shrimp Skewers

Ingredients

- Shrimp
- Cajun seasoning
- Lemon
- Olive oil
- Garlic
- Paprika

Preparation

- Toss shrimp with Cajun seasoning, lemon, olive oil, garlic, and paprika.
- Put on skewers and cook under the grill until done.

Nutritional Information

- Calories: 200
- Protein: 20g
- Carbohydrates: 5g
- Fat: 10g

Serving Size: 4 skewers

Preparation Time: 15 minutes

9. Halibut with Roasted Vegetables
Ingredients

- Halibut fillets
- Zucchini
- Cherry tomatoes
- Bell peppers
- Red onion
- Olive oil
- Italian herbs
- Garlic
- Lemon

Preparation

- Place halibut fillets on a bed of zucchini, cherry tomatoes, bell peppers, and red onion.

- Drizzle with olive oil, sprinkle with Italian herbs, garlic, and lemon.
- Roast until fish is flaky.

Nutritional Information

- Calories: 280
- Protein: 30g
- Carbohydrates: 15g
- Fat: 12g
- Fiber: 5g

Serving Size: 1 fillet with vegetables

Preparation Time: 35 minutes

10. Seared Scallops with Lemon Butter Sauce

Ingredients

- Scallops
- Lemon
- Butter
- Garlic
- Parsley
- Salt, pepper

Preparation

- Sear scallops in a hot pan with lemon, butter, garlic, parsley, salt, and pepper until golden brown.

Nutritional Information

- Calories: 200
- Protein: 20g
- Carbohydrates: 5g
- Fat: 10g

Serving Size: 4 ounces

Preparation Time: 15 minutes

CHAPTER 8

Main Dish- Vegetarian

1. Eggplant and Chickpea Curry

Ingredients

- Eggplant
- Chickpeas
- Tomatoes
- Onion
- Garlic
- Ginger
- Coconut milk
- Curry powder, salt, pepper, turmeric, cumin, and coriander

Preparation

- Sauté onion, garlic, and ginger.
- Add eggplant, chickpeas, tomatoes, coconut milk, and spices.
- Simmer until flavors meld.

Nutritional Information

- Calories: 280
- Protein: 10g
- Carbohydrates: 35g
- Dietary Fiber: 12g

Serving Size: 1.5 cups

Preparation Time: 35 minutes

2. Mushroom and Spinach Risotto

Ingredients

- Arborio rice
- Mushrooms
- Spinach
- Vegetable broth
- Onion
- Garlic
- Parmesan cheese
- Olive oil

- White wine (optional)
- Salt, pepper

Preparation

- Sauté onion and garlic, add mushrooms and spinach.
- Stir in Arborio rice, add vegetable broth gradually, and cook until creamy.
- Finish with Parmesan.

Nutritional Information

- Calories: 320
- Protein: 10g
- Carbohydrates: 45g
- Dietary Fiber: 5g

Serving Size: 1 cup

Preparation Time: 40 minutes

3. Sweet Potato and Black Bean Enchiladas

Ingredients

- Sweet potatoes
- Black beans
- Corn tortillas
- Enchilada sauce
- Red onion
- Cilantro
- Lime juice
- Cumin, chili powder, salt, pepper

Preparation

- Roast sweet potatoes, mix with black beans, red onion, cilantro, lime juice, and spices. Fill tortillas, roll, and top with enchilada sauce. Bake until bubbly.

Nutritional Information

- Calories: 300
- Protein: 10g
- Carbohydrates: 50g
- Dietary Fiber: 12g

Serving Size: 2 enchiladas

Preparation Time: 45 minutes

4. Quinoa and Vegetable Stir-Fry

Ingredients

- Quinoa
- Broccoli
- Bell peppers
- Carrots
- Snap peas
- Soy sauce
- Ginger
- Garlic
- Olive oil
- Sesame seeds

Preparation

- Cook quinoa, stir-fry vegetables in olive oil, add soy sauce, ginger, and garlic.
- Mix with quinoa and sprinkle with sesame seeds.

Nutritional Information

- Calories: 280
- Protein: 12g
- Carbohydrates: 40g
- Dietary Fiber: 8g

Serving Size: 1.5 cups

Preparation Time: 30 minutes

5. Caprese Quinoa Salad

Ingredients

- Quinoa
- Cherry tomatoes
- Mozzarella balls
- Fresh basil
- Balsamic vinegar
- Olive oil
- Salt, pepper

Preparation

- Cook quinoa, mix with halved cherry tomatoes, mozzarella balls, and fresh basil.
- Drizzle with olive oil and balsamic vinegar.
- Season with salt and pepper.

Nutritional Information

- Calories: 250
- Protein: 10g
- Carbohydrates: 30g
- Dietary Fiber: 5g

Serving Size: 1.5 cups

Preparation Time: 25 minutes

6. Chickpea and Vegetable Curry

Ingredients

- Chickpeas
- Cauliflower
- Bell peppers
- Tomatoes
- Onion
- Garlic
- Ginger
- Coconut milk

- Turmeric, cumin, coriander, curry powder, salt, and pepper

Preparation

- Sauté onion, garlic, and ginger.
- Add chickpeas, cauliflower, bell peppers, tomatoes, coconut milk, and spices.
- Simmer until flavors meld.

Nutritional Information

- Calories: 320
- Protein: 14g
- Carbohydrates: 40g
- Dietary Fiber: 12g

Serving Size: 1.5 cups

Preparation Time: 35 minutes

7. Stuffed Bell Peppers with Quinoa and Black Beans

Ingredients

- Bell peppers
- Quinoa
- Black beans
- Corn
- Tomatoes
- Onion
- Garlic
- Cumin, chili powder, salt, pepper

Preparation

- Cook quinoa, mix with black beans, corn, tomatoes, onion, garlic, and spices.
- Stuff bell peppers and bake until tender.

Nutritional Information

- Calories: 280
- Protein: 12g

- Carbohydrates: 45g
- Dietary Fiber: 10g

Serving Size: 2 stuffed peppers

Preparation Time: 40 minutes

8. Pesto Zucchini Noodles with Cherry Tomatoes

Ingredients

- Zucchini noodles
- Cherry tomatoes
- Pesto sauce
- Pine nuts
- Parmesan cheese
- Olive oil
- Garlic
- Salt, pepper

Preparation

- Sauté zucchini noodles in olive oil with cherry tomatoes, garlic, and pesto sauce.
- Top with toasted pine nuts and Parmesan.

Nutritional Information

- Calories: 220
- Protein: 5g
- Carbohydrates: 15g
- Dietary Fiber: 4g

Serving Size: 1.5 cups

Preparation Time: 20 minutes

CHAPTER 9

Conclusion

The aim of creating this cookbook for those enduring chemotherapy was to provide more than just recipes, but also a supportive culinary guidance for such a difficult journey. Navigating the delicate balance of diet throughout chemotherapy necessitates knowledge, adaptation, and a dedication to promoting overall health.

Each food in this cookbook has been carefully crafted to meet the specific needs of people undergoing chemotherapy. Our recipes stress the healing power of healthy foods, with protein-packed dishes that aid in tissue regeneration, fiber-rich meals that support digestive health, and antioxidant-rich foods that contribute to cellular defense.

We recognize that taste preferences, appetites, and nutritional tolerances may change during this time. Therefore, flexibility is crucial. The emphasis is not only on what to eat, but also on developing a healthy relationship with food. Whether you like the comfort of a warm soup or the simplicity of a smoothie, our recipes are intended to bring both sustenance and enjoyment.

Keep in mind that your culinary adventure will be unique to you. Consultation with healthcare specialists or qualified dietitians is recommended to adjust dietary choices to individual needs and treatment regimens. This cookbook is a helpful companion, providing inspiration and practical advice, but maintaining your health is a team effort.

May these recipes not only nourish your body, but also provide you joy and fulfillment. Here's to a nourishing chemo journey that considers both physical and emotional well-being. Stay strong, appreciate every mouthful, and know that you are not alone on this healing journey.

I wish you strength, nourishment, and comfort.

Printed in Great Britain
by Amazon